DIFFICULTY ACHIEVING ORGASM "ANORGASMIA"

Knowing The Causes And Permanent Solution To Anorgasmia; The Inability To Achieve Orgasm Despite Enough Stimulation

Dr. Arthur Myles

Copyright©2025 Dr. Arthur Myles
All Right Reserved

TABLE OF CONTENTS

INTRODUCTION TO ANORGASMIA _____ 4
  Prevalence and Impact _____ 5

CHAPTER 1 _____ 8
  Causes of Anorgasmia _____ 8
    Psychological Factors _____ 8
    Physical Factors _____ 10
    Physical Injury or Surgery _____ 12
    Age-Related Factors _____ 13
    Lack of Knowledge or Experience __ 14

CHAPTER 2 _____ 16
  Symptoms and Diagnosis _____ 16
    When to Seek Professional Help __ 24

CHAPTER 3 _____ 26
  Permanent Solutions to Anorgasmia 26

CHAPTER 4 _____ 40
  Natural Solutions to Anorgasmia __ 40

CHAPTER 5 _____ 54

CHAPTER 6 _____ 70
  Conclusion _____ 70
    Moving Forward with Solutions __ 72

Importance of Professional Guidance _____73

INTRODUCTION TO ANORGASMIA

Anorgasmia, also known as the inability to achieve orgasm, is a condition in which a person cannot reach orgasm despite sufficient sexual stimulation. It is a form of sexual dysfunction that can affect both men and women, though it tends to be more common among women. Anorgasmia can have a significant impact on a person's sexual health, emotional well-being, and intimate relationships.

Orgasm is a complex physiological and psychological process that involves the nervous system, hormones, and emotional factors. Achieving orgasm typically requires the right combination of physical stimulation, emotional arousal, and mental focus. When this process is disrupted in some way, it may result in anorgasmia.

Prevalence and Impact

Anorgasmia is more common than many people realize. Studies suggest that between 10% and 40% of women and about 5% of men experience some form of anorgasmia at some point in their lives. The condition can occur at any stage of life, whether a person has previously experienced orgasms or never reached orgasm at all.

The impact of anorgasmia can be profound, affecting an individual's self-esteem, relationships, and overall quality of life. People may experience feelings of frustration, disappointment, or shame, and this can create tension or conflict in intimate relationships. For some, the inability to achieve orgasm may cause emotional distress or contribute to anxiety and depression.

While anorgasmia can be temporary or situational, for others, it may be a chronic issue requiring professional intervention and treatment.

Understanding the causes and solutions for anorgasmia is crucial in helping individuals regain control over their sexual health and enhance their overall sense of well-being.

CHAPTER 1

Causes of Anorgasmia

Anorgasmia can result from a variety of physical, psychological, and relational factors. Identifying the underlying causes is essential in determining the most effective approach to treatment. Below are the primary causes of anorgasmia:

Psychological Factors
Stress and Anxiety
High levels of stress, especially performance anxiety related to sex, can interfere with the ability to achieve orgasm. Anxiety can distract

the mind, making it difficult to focus on physical sensations and arousal.

Depression

Depression can significantly impact libido and sexual function. Feelings of sadness, low energy, and a lack of interest in pleasurable activities often diminish sexual drive and the ability to experience orgasm.

Trauma and Abuse

Past experiences of sexual trauma or abuse can create psychological blocks to sexual pleasure. Individuals may struggle with feelings of fear, shame, or mistrust, which hinder their ability to fully relax and enjoy sexual activity, preventing orgasm.

Relationship Issues

Poor communication, emotional distance, unresolved conflicts, or lack of intimacy with a partner can contribute to anorgasmia. Without a strong sense of emotional connection and trust, it can be challenging to achieve sexual satisfaction.

Physical Factors
Hormonal Imbalances

Hormonal fluctuations or imbalances, particularly in estrogen, progesterone, and testosterone, can affect libido and orgasm. Menopause, pregnancy, or the use of birth control can result in hormonal changes that impact sexual function.

Neurological Conditions

Diseases or conditions that affect the nervous system, such as multiple sclerosis, diabetes, or spinal cord injuries, can disrupt the nerve pathways responsible for sexual response and orgasm.

Chronic Illnesses and Medical Conditions

Chronic conditions like diabetes, cardiovascular disease, and high blood pressure can affect circulation, nerve function, and overall sexual health.

These conditions may contribute to decreased sensitivity or difficulty reaching orgasm.

Medications and Substance Use
Some medications, especially antidepressants (e.g., SSRIs), antihypertensives, and birth control pills, can cause side effects that hinder sexual arousal and orgasm. Alcohol, drugs, and smoking also negatively impact sexual function and orgasmic ability.

Physical Injury or Surgery
Pelvic Injury
Injuries to the pelvic region, such as from accidents, surgery, or trauma,

can damage the nerves or disrupt blood flow, making orgasm difficult or impossible.

Childbirth-Related Changes

After childbirth, especially in cases of difficult delivery or episiotomy, women may experience physical changes that affect the pelvic floor and genital sensitivity. These changes may hinder sexual pleasure and the ability to achieve orgasm.

Age-Related Factors
Age-Related Changes

As individuals age, physical and hormonal changes occur that can affect sexual function. In women, menopause and decreased estrogen levels can lead to vaginal dryness, reduced sensitivity, and difficulty achieving orgasm. In men, lower testosterone levels may reduce sexual desire and the ability to orgasm.

Lack of Knowledge or Experience
Inexperience or Lack of Sexual Education
Individuals who lack sexual experience or do not fully understand their own bodies may struggle to identify the types of stimulation that lead to orgasm. A lack of sexual knowledge or exposure to various sexual activities can limit the ability to reach orgasm.

Decreased Sexual Pleasure

Many individuals with anorgasmia report a decrease in the overall enjoyment of sexual activity, even if they experience arousal or physical pleasure during sex.

Frustration or Distress

The inability to orgasm can lead to feelings of frustration, disappointment, or inadequacy. This emotional distress can exacerbate the problem, creating a cycle of anxiety or tension around sex.

Reduced Libido or Desire

Some individuals with anorgasmia may experience a decrease in sexual desire or interest, as the lack of orgasm can make sex feel less rewarding.

Difficulty Achieving Orgasm in Specific Situations

In some cases, anorgasmia may occur only in certain situations, such as with specific partners or sexual activities. For example, someone may be able to orgasm during masturbation but not during intercourse, or vice versa.

Physical Changes During Sexual Activity

Even when aroused, a person with anorgasmia may experience reduced vaginal or penile sensitivity, which can contribute to difficulty in reaching orgasm.

Diagnosis of Anorgasmia

The diagnosis of anorgasmia typically involves a comprehensive evaluation by a healthcare provider, often a gynecologist, urologist, or sex therapist. A thorough assessment is necessary to rule out any underlying physical or psychological causes. The diagnostic process typically includes the following steps:

Medical History Review

The healthcare provider will gather a detailed medical history, including information about past sexual experiences, menstrual or reproductive history (for women), and any existing medical conditions. This information helps identify potential physical causes of anorgasmia.

Psychological and Emotional Evaluation

Psychological factors, including stress, anxiety, depression, trauma, or relationship issues, are common contributors to anorgasmia. The provider may ask about mental health history, emotional well-being, and any past experiences that may be affecting sexual function.

Sexual History Assessment

The provider may ask about the person's sexual activity, including frequency of orgasm, types of stimulation that have been tried, and whether orgasm is possible during solo sexual activity (e.g., masturbation). This helps assess whether the problem is specific to partnered sex or affects all forms of sexual activity.

Physical Examination

A physical examination may be necessary to rule out underlying medical conditions or anatomical issues that could contribute to anorgasmia. For women, this may include a pelvic exam, while for men, a genital exam may be conducted to check for any abnormalities or issues with blood flow or nerve function.

Laboratory Tests

Blood tests may be recommended to check for hormonal imbalances, thyroid function, or other potential underlying medical conditions such as diabetes or other health issues that could affect sexual function.

Psychological Testing or Counseling

In cases where psychological factors like anxiety, depression, or trauma are suspected, a mental health professional may conduct assessments or therapy sessions. This could involve standardized questionnaires or counseling sessions to explore emotional barriers to sexual function.

Partner and Relationship Evaluation
Since relationship dynamics can significantly influence sexual health, the provider may suggest a couple's assessment or therapy to address any interpersonal issues affecting sexual satisfaction.

Trial of Self-Exploration or Sexual Techniques
The healthcare provider may recommend techniques such as self-exploration or specific sexual positions to see if they make a difference in achieving orgasm. These techniques help the

individual gain a better understanding of what types of stimulation or settings work best for them.

When to Seek Professional Help
Anorgasmia is not uncommon, but if the condition persists and causes emotional or relational distress, seeking professional help is important. Individuals should consider consulting a healthcare provider or therapist if:

The inability to orgasm is ongoing or affects sexual relationships.
There is emotional distress, anxiety, or depression related to sexual performance.

The condition occurs suddenly or after a significant life event, injury, or medical condition.
The person is experiencing a decrease in sexual desire or pleasure.

There are concerns about underlying medical conditions or medications contributing to the issue.
Prompt professional intervention can help identify the causes of anorgasmia and explore treatment options to improve sexual health and satisfaction.

CHAPTER 3

Permanent Solutions to Anorgasmia

Addressing anorgasmia effectively often requires a multifaceted approach, combining medical treatments, psychological support, and lifestyle adjustments. By identifying the root causes—whether psychological, physical, or relational—individuals can work toward a long-term solution to improve their sexual health and satisfaction. Below are permanent solutions to help overcome anorgasmia:

Medical Treatments

Hormone Therapy

Hormonal imbalances can contribute significantly to anorgasmia. For individuals experiencing hormonal changes (e.g., menopause or low testosterone), hormone replacement therapy (HRT) may be recommended to restore balance and improve sexual function. This may include estrogen therapy for women going through menopause or testosterone therapy for both men and women with low levels.

Medication Adjustments

Some medications, such as antidepressants (especially SSRIs) and certain antihypertensives, can negatively affect sexual function. If medications are identified as a contributing factor to anorgasmia, a healthcare provider may adjust the dosage, switch medications, or recommend alternative drugs with fewer sexual side effects. It's important not to stop any prescribed medications without consulting a doctor.

Treatment for Underlying Health Conditions

Anorgasmia may be a symptom of an underlying medical condition like diabetes, cardiovascular disease, or neurological disorders. Managing these conditions through appropriate medication, lifestyle changes, or surgery can improve overall sexual function and reduce the impact of physical health issues on orgasm.

Psychotherapy and Counseling
Cognitive Behavioral Therapy (CBT)
CBT is an effective therapeutic approach for addressing anxiety, depression, or negative thought patterns that may be contributing to anorgasmia. CBT helps individuals identify and challenge irrational beliefs and fears related to sex, promoting a healthier and more positive mindset about sexual activity.

Sex Therapy

Sex therapy with a licensed therapist can help individuals or couples explore emotional barriers to sexual satisfaction and orgasm. This therapy often includes learning about sexual techniques, communication skills, and strategies to improve intimacy and pleasure. A sex therapist may also help individuals explore their body's response to different kinds of sexual stimulation.

Trauma-Informed Therapy

For those with a history of sexual trauma or abuse, therapy focused on healing past wounds is crucial. Trauma-informed therapy helps individuals process and heal from past trauma, which can break down psychological blocks and emotional barriers that interfere with sexual function.

Couples Counseling

If relationship dynamics are contributing to anorgasmia, couples therapy can help improve communication, resolve conflicts, and rebuild intimacy. Strengthening the emotional connection between partners can create a safe and trusting environment where both individuals feel comfortable exploring and enjoying their sexual lives.

Pelvic Floor Exercises

Kegel Exercises

Kegel exercises, which involve strengthening the pelvic floor muscles, can help improve sexual arousal and orgasm, particularly in women. Strong pelvic muscles contribute to better blood flow to the genital area, increased sensitivity, and more intense orgasms. Men can also benefit from pelvic floor exercises, which help with erectile function and orgasmic control.

Pelvic Physical Therapy

A trained pelvic physical therapist can assess and treat physical issues related to the pelvic floor, such as muscle tension, weakness, or injury.

This therapy may involve manual techniques, biofeedback, or exercises to restore pelvic floor function and improve sexual satisfaction.

Lifestyle Modifications

Stress Management

Chronic stress is a significant contributor to sexual dysfunction. Adopting stress-reduction techniques such as yoga, meditation, deep breathing exercises, or mindfulness can help relax the body and mind, reducing anxiety and making it easier to focus on sexual pleasure. Regular physical activity, adequate sleep, and time for relaxation also play a vital role in managing stress.

Nutrition and Hydration

A healthy, balanced diet supports overall well-being, including sexual health. Nutrient-rich foods that promote blood circulation (e.g., fruits, vegetables, and healthy fats) and hormone balance (e.g., zinc, omega-3 fatty acids) can improve sexual function. Staying hydrated is also essential for maintaining proper blood flow and genital sensitivity.

Limiting Alcohol and Drug Use

Excessive alcohol, recreational drug use, or smoking can impair sexual function and contribute to anorgasmia. Reducing or eliminating these substances can help restore sexual health and improve the ability to reach orgasm.

Exploring New Sexual Techniques
Self-Exploration
Masturbation and self-exploration are essential tools for individuals to understand their bodies and what types of stimulation bring them the most pleasure. This practice can help people become more comfortable with their sexual responses, which can increase the chances of orgasm during partnered sex.

Communication with Partner

Open and honest communication with a sexual partner about desires, preferences, and what feels good is key to overcoming anorgasmia. Talking about sexual needs can help both partners feel more connected and lead to improved intimacy and sexual satisfaction.

Sexual Techniques and Positions

Experimenting with different sexual positions or using clitoral or other types of stimulation (e.g., vibrators or other sex toys) can enhance arousal and increase the likelihood of orgasm. For women, clitoral stimulation is often necessary to achieve orgasm, while some men may benefit from exploring different types of physical stimulation for more intense orgasms.

Alternative Therapies

Acupuncture

Acupuncture is sometimes used as an alternative treatment to enhance sexual function. It is thought to help improve blood flow, balance hormones, and address psychological blocks related to sexual pleasure. While more research is needed, some individuals find acupuncture helpful in overcoming sexual dysfunction.

Herbal Supplements

Certain herbs, like ginseng, maca root, or horny goat weed, are sometimes used to boost libido and improve sexual function. However, it's important to consult with a healthcare provider before taking any herbal supplements to ensure they are safe and effective.

Anorgasmia can often be treated successfully with a combination of medical interventions, psychotherapy, physical exercises, and lifestyle changes. A personalized approach that addresses the root causes—whether psychological, physical, or relational—can help individuals regain control over their sexual health and enjoy fulfilling sexual experiences. Seeking professional help from a healthcare provider or therapist is an important first step toward finding an effective, permanent solution for anorgasmia.

CHAPTER 4

Natural Solutions to Anorgasmia

In addition to medical treatments and psychotherapy, natural solutions can play a vital role in overcoming anorgasmia. These solutions focus on lifestyle changes, dietary adjustments, and alternative therapies that can improve sexual health and function. Below are some effective natural approaches to help address anorgasmia:

Herbal Supplements

Several herbs have been traditionally used to boost sexual health and improve libido. Some of the most popular herbs that may help with anorgasmia include:

Maca Root

Known as a natural aphrodisiac, maca root is believed to enhance sexual desire, improve energy levels, and balance hormones. Studies have suggested that maca can help improve sexual function and satisfaction in both men and women.

Ginseng

Panax ginseng is thought to improve blood flow, enhance sexual arousal, and increase sensitivity. It is commonly used as an herbal remedy to combat erectile dysfunction and enhance sexual performance, potentially improving orgasmic ability in both men and women.

Horny Goat Weed
This herb has been used in traditional Chinese medicine to treat sexual dysfunction. It is believed to increase blood flow to the genital area and may enhance sexual desire and performance. Some research suggests it can support libido and overall sexual health.

Tribulus Terrestris
This herb has been shown to help regulate testosterone levels and

improve libido. It may be particularly beneficial for those with low sexual desire due to hormonal imbalances.

Ashwagandha
Often used in Ayurvedic medicine, ashwagandha is an adaptogen that helps reduce stress and anxiety, which are often contributing factors to anorgasmia. By lowering stress levels, it can indirectly help improve sexual function.

Lifestyle Changes
Stress Reduction Techniques
High levels of stress and anxiety can inhibit the ability to achieve orgasm. Incorporating relaxation techniques

such as mindfulness, deep breathing exercises, yoga, or meditation can help reduce stress, promote emotional well-being, and create a calm mental state conducive to sexual pleasure.

Regular Exercise

Physical activity can significantly boost sexual health by improving blood circulation, reducing stress, and balancing hormones. Activities like walking, running, or yoga help maintain a healthy weight, increase energy levels, and improve overall physical function, which can positively affect sexual response.

Sleep Hygiene

Adequate rest is essential for hormonal balance and overall sexual health. Lack of sleep can negatively affect libido and sexual function. Aim for 7-9 hours of quality sleep each night to improve mood, energy levels, and sexual well-being.

Limiting Alcohol and Substance Use
Excessive alcohol consumption, smoking, and recreational drug use can impair sexual function and reduce sensitivity, making orgasm difficult to achieve. Reducing or eliminating these substances can help improve sexual response and function.

Nutrition and Diet

What you eat can have a direct impact on sexual health and orgasmic ability. Incorporating certain foods and nutrients can help enhance libido and overall sexual function.

Foods Rich in Zinc

Zinc plays a key role in hormone production, including testosterone. Foods like pumpkin seeds, shellfish, red meat, and legumes are rich in zinc and can support healthy sexual function.

Omega-3 Fatty Acids

Omega-3 fatty acids, found in foods like salmon, flaxseeds, and walnuts, improve blood circulation, which is essential for arousal and orgasm. Omega-3s may also help balance hormones and reduce inflammation in the body.

Dark Chocolate

Dark chocolate contains compounds that increase serotonin and endorphin levels in the brain, promoting feelings of pleasure and well-being. It may also improve blood flow, which can enhance sexual function.

Leafy Greens and Beets

Vegetables such as spinach, kale, and beets are rich in nitrates, which help increase blood flow by relaxing blood vessels. Improved circulation to the genital area is crucial for achieving orgasm.

Water and Hydration
Staying hydrated is important for overall health, including sexual health. Proper hydration ensures optimal circulation, genital sensitivity, and energy levels, all of which contribute to the ability to orgasm.

Pelvic Floor Exercises
Strengthening the pelvic floor muscles can improve sexual function and increase the likelihood of orgasm. These muscles are responsible for the sensations experienced during orgasm,

so enhancing their strength and control can be beneficial.

Kegel Exercises

Kegel exercises involve contracting and relaxing the pelvic floor muscles. These exercises can increase sexual pleasure by enhancing muscle tone, improving blood flow, and boosting sensitivity in the genital area. Both men and women can benefit from Kegel exercises.

Pelvic Physical Therapy

For individuals with pelvic floor dysfunction (such as tension or weakness), seeing a pelvic floor therapist can be an excellent way to improve muscle function. This therapy includes exercises, manual techniques, and biofeedback to enhance pelvic muscle control and improve orgasmic ability.

Acupuncture and Acupressure

Acupuncture is a form of traditional Chinese medicine that involves inserting thin needles into specific points on the body. It is believed to help restore balance in the body and improve energy flow (known as "qi").

Acupuncture

Acupuncture has been used to treat sexual dysfunction by increasing blood flow, balancing hormones, and reducing stress. Some studies have suggested that acupuncture can help with issues like anorgasmia by enhancing sexual arousal and response.

Acupressure

Acupressure is a less invasive alternative to acupuncture that involves applying pressure to specific points on the body. Some people find that acupressure helps with reducing stress, enhancing sexual pleasure, and addressing physical blockages that may interfere with orgasm.

Mind-Body Practices

Mindfulness and Meditation

Mindfulness is the practice of being fully present in the moment without judgment. It can improve sexual experiences by reducing mental distractions, helping individuals connect more deeply with their bodies and partners during sex. Meditation techniques can also be used to reduce anxiety and improve sexual awareness and response.

Tantric Practices
Tantra is a spiritual practice that focuses on deep connection and mindfulness during sex. Incorporating tantric techniques into sexual activity may enhance orgasm by promoting relaxation, breathing

techniques, and emotional intimacy with a partner.

Natural solutions to anorgasmia often focus on lifestyle changes, stress management, nutrition, physical exercises, and alternative therapies that support overall sexual health. By integrating these practices into daily life, individuals may experience improved sexual function, greater pleasure, and the ability to achieve orgasm. However, it's important to approach these solutions in combination with professional medical advice, especially if the issue is chronic or associated with an underlying medical condition.

CHAPTER 5

Prevention and Long-Term Management

While anorgasmia can occur due to a variety of factors, it is possible to take proactive steps to prevent its onset and manage it over the long term. By focusing on lifestyle, emotional well-being, communication, and sexual health, individuals can maintain optimal sexual function and prevent recurring issues with orgasm.

Prioritize Emotional and Mental Health

Manage Stress and Anxiety

Chronic stress and anxiety are significant contributors to sexual dysfunction, including anorgasmia.

Regular practice of stress-reduction techniques such as yoga, deep breathing, meditation, and mindfulness can help maintain emotional well-being and reduce the mental barriers to orgasm. Managing anxiety, particularly performance anxiety, can significantly improve sexual satisfaction.

Address Depression and Negative Emotions
Ongoing feelings of sadness, guilt, or inadequacy can also interfere with sexual function. Seeking therapy or counseling to address depression, self-esteem issues, or past trauma can help individuals develop a healthier

mindset and a more positive relationship with their bodies and sexuality. Cognitive behavioral therapy (CBT) is often effective in changing negative thought patterns that contribute to sexual dysfunction.

Engage in Relationship Counseling
Open communication and emotional intimacy between partners are essential for sexual well-being. Couples should prioritize building trust, resolving conflicts, and nurturing emotional closeness. Regular relationship counseling or sex therapy can help address issues related to sexual satisfaction and

prevent relational factors from affecting orgasm.

Maintain a Healthy Lifestyle

Regular Exercise

Regular physical activity is crucial for overall health and well-being. Exercise improves circulation, boosts energy levels, reduces stress, and helps balance hormones, all of which are vital for sexual health. Cardiovascular exercises (e.g., walking, running, cycling) and strength training can promote better blood flow, which is essential for sexual arousal and orgasm.

Balanced Diet and Nutrition

Eating a nutrient-rich diet supports healthy sexual function. Focus on consuming whole foods, including fruits, vegetables, lean proteins, and healthy fats, to improve circulation and hormonal balance. Include foods rich in zinc (e.g., pumpkin seeds, shellfish), omega-3 fatty acids (e.g., salmon, flaxseeds), and antioxidants (e.g., berries, dark chocolate) to support sexual health. Staying hydrated is also critical for maintaining good circulation and energy levels.

Avoid Excessive Alcohol and Drug Use Alcohol and recreational drugs can impair sexual function and contribute to difficulties achieving orgasm. Limiting alcohol consumption and avoiding recreational drugs and smoking can help ensure sexual function remains optimal. If alcohol or drug use is a factor in anorgasmia, reducing or eliminating these substances can significantly improve sexual health.

Quality Sleep

Sleep is essential for overall health, including sexual well-being. Chronic sleep deprivation can lead to hormonal imbalances, fatigue, and decreased libido. Aim for 7-9 hours of uninterrupted sleep each night to support your physical and mental health, as well as your sexual function.

Regular Health Check-ups

Monitor Hormonal Health

Hormonal imbalances, particularly during periods of significant life changes (e.g., menopause, aging, or after childbirth), can impact sexual function. Regular health check-ups can help detect any hormonal imbalances that may affect libido and orgasm. If needed, hormone replacement therapy (HRT) or other interventions can be considered to help restore hormonal balance and improve sexual health.

Manage Chronic Conditions

Chronic health conditions such as diabetes, cardiovascular disease, or neurological disorders can contribute to sexual dysfunction. Keeping chronic conditions under control through regular medical check-ups, medication, and lifestyle modifications can help prevent sexual health issues from affecting orgasmic ability.

Medication Review
If you are taking medications that might impact sexual function (e.g., antidepressants, birth control pills, or antihypertensives), review these with your healthcare provider. They may suggest alternative medications

with fewer sexual side effects. Always consult your doctor before making any changes to your medication regimen.

Practice Communication and Connection with Partners

Open Communication About Sexual Needs

One of the most effective ways to prevent and manage anorgasmia is through open, honest communication with your partner about your sexual needs, desires, and preferences. Discussing what feels good, what might be inhibiting orgasm, and any areas of discomfort can help foster emotional intimacy and create a supportive environment for sexual exploration.

Explore Intimacy Beyond Orgasm

It's important to remember that sexual intimacy does not solely revolve around achieving orgasm. Focusing on the overall experience of pleasure, connection, and shared intimacy with your partner can reduce pressure and anxiety related to orgasm. Exploring different forms of physical touch, such as cuddling, kissing, or sensual massages, can help deepen emotional connection and enhance sexual satisfaction.

Engage in Regular Physical Affection

Maintaining physical closeness and affection outside of sexual activity helps build emotional trust and intimacy, creating a supportive foundation for a fulfilling sexual relationship. Regular affection (holding hands, hugging, kissing) can also help alleviate stress and promote a positive relationship with your partner.

Self-Exploration and Sexual Awareness
Explore Your Body and Sexual Preferences
Understanding your own body and what gives you pleasure is an essential step in overcoming anorgasmia. Regular self-exploration through masturbation can help you discover the types of stimulation that work best for you, whether clitoral, vaginal, or a

combination of both. Increased awareness of your sexual preferences and needs can help guide sexual experiences with a partner and improve orgasmic potential.

Incorporate Mindfulness and Focus on Sensations

Being present during sexual activity can help you connect more deeply with your body and sexual responses. Mindfulness techniques, such as focusing on physical sensations and deep breathing, can reduce mental distractions, increase awareness of pleasure, and support the ability to achieve orgasm.

Experiment with Different Techniques and Positions

Trying new sexual techniques, positions, or forms of stimulation can help identify what works best for you and your partner. It's important to maintain an open mind and communicate with your partner to ensure both of your needs are met during sexual activity.

Addressing Psychological and Emotional Barriers

Therapy for Trauma or Past Negative Experiences

If past trauma or negative sexual experiences are contributing to anorgasmia, seeking therapy can help address emotional barriers to sexual function. Trauma-informed therapy can help individuals work through feelings of shame, guilt, or fear, and provide tools for overcoming psychological blocks related to sex.

Consider Sex Therapy

Sex therapy with a licensed therapist can help individuals or couples address emotional or psychological issues related to sexuality. Sex therapists can provide guidance on improving intimacy, exploring sexual desires, and overcoming performance anxiety, leading to a more fulfilling and enjoyable sex life.

Prevention and long-term management of anorgasmia involve a comprehensive approach that includes emotional, physical, and relational well-being. By focusing on stress management, maintaining a healthy lifestyle, staying on top of medical health, and fostering open communication with partners, individuals can prevent or manage anorgasmia effectively. Incorporating self-awareness and exploring emotional and psychological factors can also help individuals achieve and maintain a fulfilling and orgasmic sexual experience. Regular check-ups with healthcare providers ensure that physical and hormonal health is maintained, and seeking therapy when needed can help overcome any psychological barriers to sexual function.

CHAPTER 6

Conclusion

Anorgasmia, the inability to achieve orgasm despite adequate sexual stimulation, can be a complex and frustrating condition that affects individuals in various ways. Its causes can be rooted in physical, psychological, or relational factors, and finding effective solutions requires a comprehensive approach that addresses these underlying causes. Whether the issue is temporary or persistent, it is important to recognize that anorgasmia is treatable, and long-term management is possible.

By incorporating natural solutions like stress management, pelvic exercises, healthy nutrition, and communication with partners, individuals can make strides toward overcoming anorgasmia. Additionally, seeking professional guidance from medical providers, therapists, or sex experts ensures that any underlying physical or psychological issues are properly diagnosed and treated. Effective treatments, such as hormone therapy, therapy for emotional or relational issues, and tailored medical interventions, can significantly improve sexual satisfaction and overall well-being.

Moving Forward with Solutions
Taking proactive steps to address anorgasmia involves understanding its causes, being open to treatment options, and engaging in regular self-care practices. For many, overcoming anorgasmia may involve a combination of lifestyle changes, emotional healing, and professional support. Moving forward with solutions requires commitment, patience, and a willingness to explore both physical and emotional dimensions of sexual health.

It's also important to remember that sexual well-being is an ongoing journey. While achieving orgasm may be the primary goal for some, fostering a fulfilling and intimate sexual connection with yourself or a partner is just as important. Emphasizing overall sexual satisfaction and emotional closeness can provide lasting fulfillment, regardless of whether orgasm is consistently achieved.

Importance of Professional Guidance
Seeking professional guidance is key to navigating the complexities of anorgasmia and finding lasting solutions. A healthcare provider,

therapist, or sex expert can help identify the root causes of the issue and recommend personalized treatments based on the individual's specific needs. Medical professionals can assess hormonal levels, treat underlying conditions, and suggest medications or therapies that may improve sexual function. Psychologists or sex therapists can help address psychological or relational factors, providing a safe and supportive space to work through issues like anxiety, trauma, or communication difficulties.

Furthermore, working with a professional ensures that any

treatments or interventions are appropriate and safe for your individual health profile. Professional guidance is particularly important if anorgasmia is causing significant distress, negatively affecting relationships, or if there is difficulty identifying the underlying causes of the issue.

By collaborating with healthcare providers and therapists, individuals can achieve a clearer understanding of their sexual health, explore effective treatment options, and work toward lasting solutions for anorgasmia. The support of a professional is an essential step in moving forward with confidence and achieving improved sexual well-being.

Made in the USA
Columbia, SC
29 May 2025